GO FACTS **HEALTHY BODIES**

Fitness

Susan Mansfield

A & C BLACK • LONDON

Fitness

contents

© 2007 Blake Publishing
Additional material © A & C Black Publishers Ltd 2009

First published in Australia by Blake Education Pty Ltd.

This edition published in the United Kingdom in 2009 by
A & C Black Publishers Ltd, 36 Soho Square, London, W1D 3QY.
www.acblack.com

Hardback edition
ISBN 978-1-4081-1227-4

Paperback edition
ISBN 978-1-4081-1223-6

A CIP record for this book is available from the British Library.

Written by Susan Mansfield
Publisher: Katy Pike
Editor: Mark Stafford
Design and layout by The Modern Art Production Group.

Printed in China by WKT Company Ltd.

Image credits: p11 bottom left — NASA

This book is produced using paper that is made from wood grown in managed
sustainable forests. It is natural, renewable and recyclable. The logging and
manufacturing processes conform to the environmental regulations of the
country of origin.

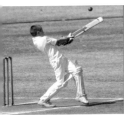

What is Fitness?

Fitness is the body's ability to be active. It consists of stamina, strength and flexibility.

Stamina

Stamina is how long a person can continue exercising. **Aerobic** exercise, such as walking, swimming, running and dancing, increases stamina. This type of exercise has repetitive actions that use the same muscle groups for at least 15 minutes.

Strength

Muscle strength comes from **anaerobic** exercise. This type of exercise uses muscles at a fast rate for a short period. It prepares the body for when it needs bursts of speed. Examples of anaerobic exercise are sprinting and weight-lifting.

Flexibility

Flexibility is the body's capacity for a full range of movements without pain. A person may have good flexibility in one joint, but be limited in another. Muscles weaken when movement is limited.

Poor flexibility of the back and hips leads to poor posture, back pain, and a higher risk of injury. Stretching and yoga are good ways to maintain flexibility.

GO FACT!

THE MOST PUSH-UPS

Japan's Minoru Yoshida did 10 507 continuous push-ups.

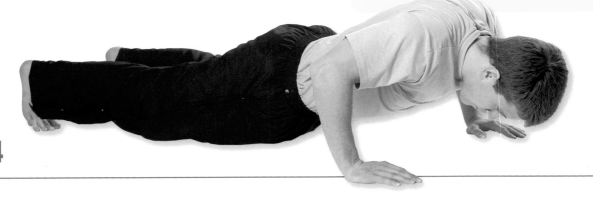

Dancing increases stamina, tones muscles and improves flexibility.

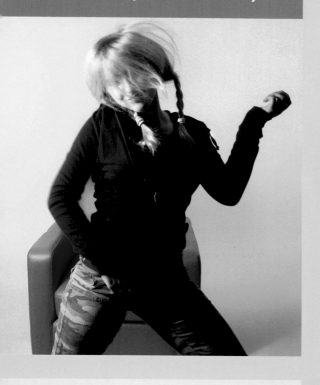

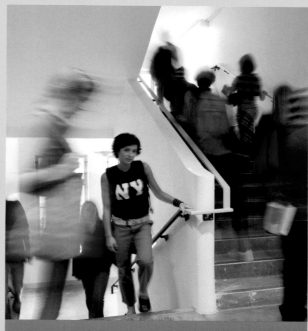

The average British student walks more than 10 000 steps each day.

Yoga was developed in India more than 5 000 years ago.

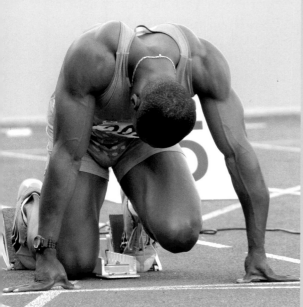

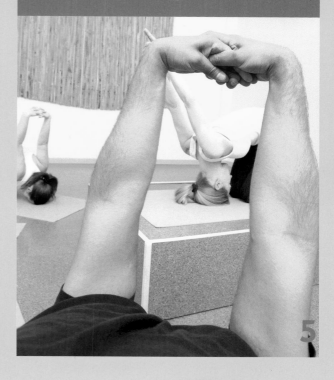

At the start of a race, sprinters need quick reflexes and explosive muscle power.

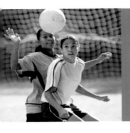

Exercise

Regular exercise improves fitness in the following ways.

Cardiovascular endurance – the ability to exercise longer and harder. The heart becomes stronger, supplying the muscles with more blood. For example, the heart rate of an 11 year-old football player rises from about 70 beats per minute before a game to above 170 beats per minute during a game.

Muscular strength – the ability to produce power for a short period. Muscles respond to use and disuse. They get bigger when they are exercised, and shrink when not used. Halil Mutlu, a Turkish weight-lifter, is 1·5 metres tall and weighs only 56 kilograms, but he can lift three times his weight above his head.

Muscular endurance – the ability to perform repeated movements without getting tired. Climbing stairs builds both muscular strength and endurance.

Flexibility – the ability of joints to move through their full, normal range of movements. Muscles that grow too large may decrease a joint's ability to move properly.

Balance – the ability to control the body's position, whether it is still or moving. Platform diving and gymnastics are both sports that require good balance.

Speed – being able to react and move quickly. Speed is important in most sports.

People between 12 and 18 years old should do at least 60 minutes of moderate to vigorous physical activity every day to stay healthy.

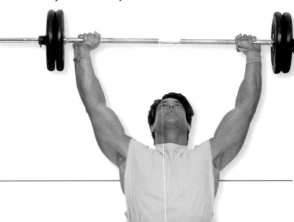

Most sports require a combination of strength, endurance, flexibility, balance and speed.

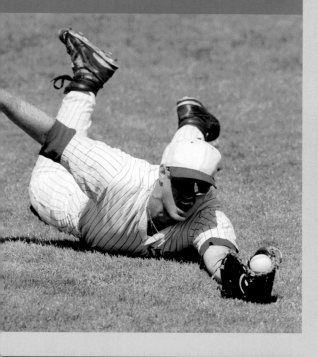

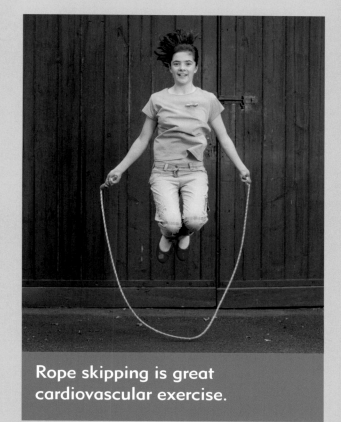

Rope skipping is great cardiovascular exercise.

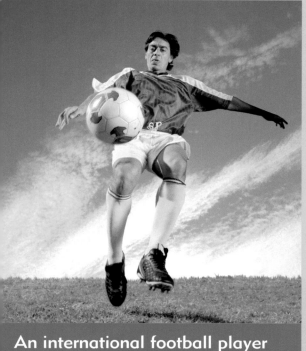

An international football player runs about 6.2 miles during a match.

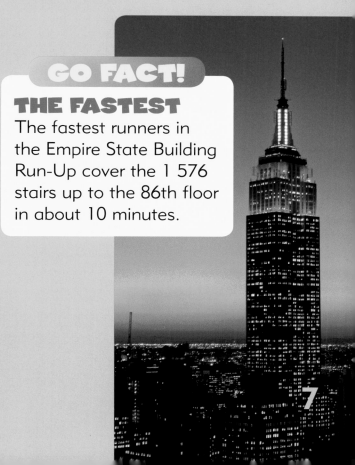

GO FACT!

THE FASTEST

The fastest runners in the Empire State Building Run-Up cover the 1 576 stairs up to the 86th floor in about 10 minutes.

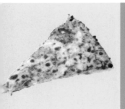

What Affects Fitness?

Fitness is affected by diet, quality of sleep and how people spend their leisure time.

Diet

An active person needs a diet that provides enough fuel for physical activity, and the **nutrients** needed for good health. This means a balanced diet of the five food groups – bread and cereals, fruit, vegetables, meat and dairy products.

Water is also important. The body can't store water and needs a fresh supply every day. Most of that water comes from the food and drink in a normal diet, but it is important to drink tap-water as well. Active people need extra water, to replace what is loss through **perspiration**.

Sleep

The amount and quality of sleep affects the body's energy levels. Teenagers need as much sleep as small children (about 10 hours each day). People over 65 years of age only need about six hours. An average adult needs eight hours of sleep each day.

Sleep also helps the body recover from exercise. Athletes often sleep in the middle of a training day to help their muscles recover.

Technology

Using computers, televisions and video games reduces how often people exercise. Leisure time is often spent sitting still, rather then being active. British children spend one-third of their leisure time watching television.

GO FACT!

DID YOU KNOW?

Runner Alberto Salazar produced 3·7 litres of sweat per hour during the 1984 Olympic marathon.

Water cushions organs and joints, and helps the body convert food into energy.

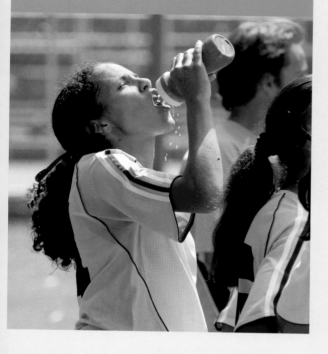

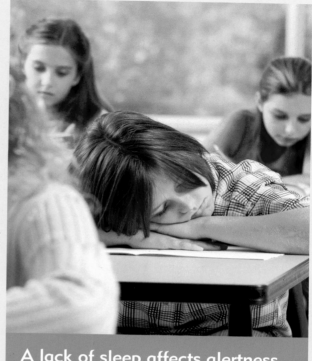

A lack of sleep affects alertness, mood and physical performance.

In a balanced diet, most food should come from fruit, vegetables, bread and cereals.

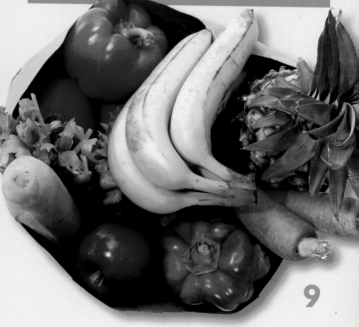

About 40 per cent of Europeans, 60 per cent of Americans and 53 per cent of Australians regularly play computer and video games.

9

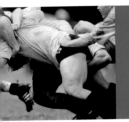

Muscles

Our bones are covered in muscles, which allow our bodies to move.

There are more than 600 **skeletal muscles** in the body. Each muscle is attached to bones by tendons, which are strong, white bands of **tissue**.

The place where two or more bones meet is called a joint. Some joints do not move, such as those in the cranium. Some joints only move slightly, such as those in the spine. Other joints move freely, such as the knee and elbow.

How muscles work

To lift a drink to your mouth, the nervous system sends a message to the biceps muscle in your upper arm. This makes the muscle contract, getting shorter and thicker. It pulls the bones of your lower arm towards your upper arm, and lifts your hand towards your mouth.

Muscles are arranged in groups. For example, the hamstring group consists of three muscles at the back of the thigh. They connect the hip bone to the shin bone (tibia).

Muscle groups often work in pairs. To produce movement, one group contracts while another relaxes. For example, to bend the knee the muscles at the back of the thigh contract and those on the front relax and stretch.

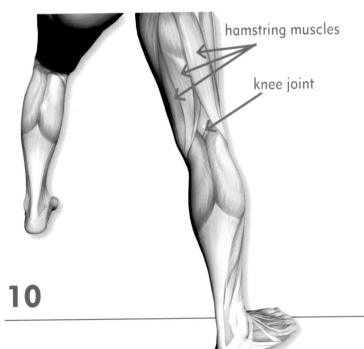

hamstring muscles

knee joint

Muscle takes up less space in the body than fat tissue. Two people of the same height and weight may have very different body shapes because of the different amounts of muscle and fat in their bodies.

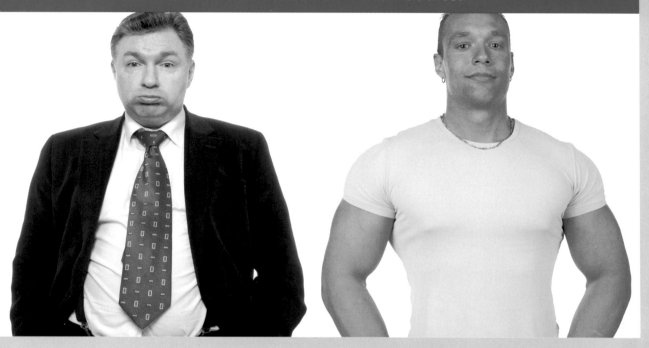

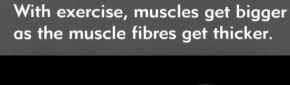
With exercise, muscles get bigger as the muscle fibres get thicker.

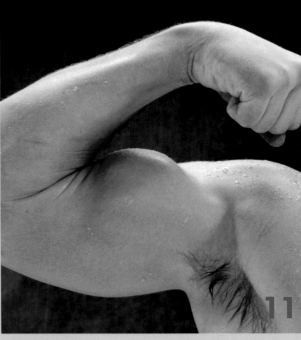

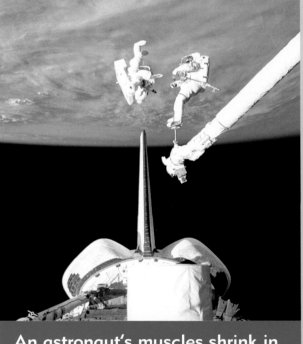
An astronaut's muscles shrink in space because they don't have to work against gravity.

11

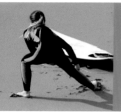

Warming up muscles lessens the chance of injury. Cooling down reduces soreness the next day.

Warming up

A warm-up routine prepares the body for exercise by increasing blood flow to muscles. It also increases the body's temperature, and heart and breathing rates.

Warm-up routines usually include a slow version of the exercise about to be done. A sprint cyclist may ride for two hours to warm up for a race that only lasts 10 minutes.

Stretching makes joints more flexible. Warming up **ligaments** makes them more **elastic** and the joint more flexible.

Cooling down

A cool-down routine helps the body clear lactic acid, a chemical that builds up in muscles during exercise. Less lactic acid means less soreness the next day.

The best way to cool down is to continue the exercise at a slower pace. Because exercise shortens muscles, stretching after physical activity is important to lengthen muscles and prevent stiffness.

A cool-down routine for a 5 000 metre running race might be slow jogging for 2–4 kilometres, and 15 minutes of stretching muscles in the legs, buttocks and back.

GO FACT!
DID YOU KNOW?

Muscles are made of 75 per cent protein, 20 per cent water, and 5 per cent salts, sugars and fat.

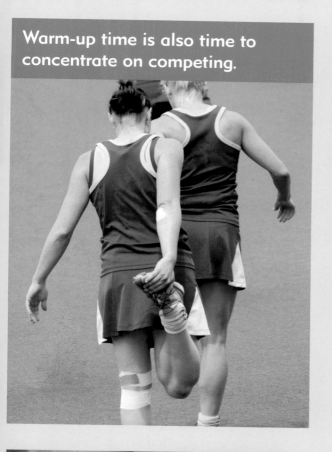

Warm-up time is also time to concentrate on competing.

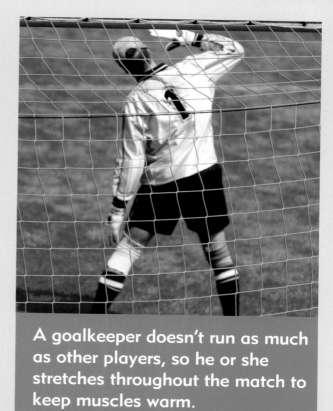

A goalkeeper doesn't run as much as other players, so he or she stretches throughout the match to keep muscles warm.

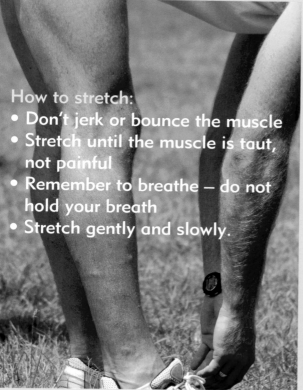

How to stretch:
- Don't jerk or bounce the muscle
- Stretch until the muscle is taut, not painful
- Remember to breathe – do not hold your breath
- Stretch gently and slowly.

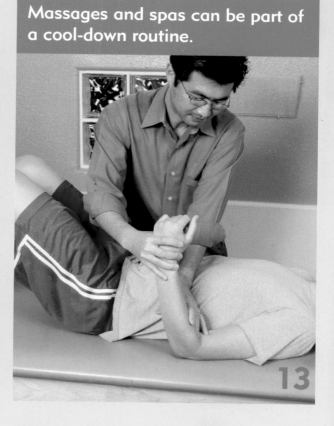

Massages and spas can be part of a cool-down routine.

13

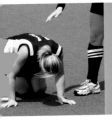

Muscle Injuries

Most fitness-related injuries are caused by exercising cold muscles or overworking them.

Muscle fibres tear when a muscle is strained. The muscle bleeds for 24–48 hours and becomes **inflamed**. Tendons and ligaments may also tear. A torn ligament is called a sprain.

There are three levels of muscle injury.

Grade 1 – Mild

Up to half the muscle's fibres are damaged. There is some swelling and pain. The injury requires a 2–3 week recovery.

Grade 2 – Moderate

More than half the muscle's fibres are damaged. There is bleeding and loss of strength. The injury requires a 3–5 week recovery.

Grade 3 – Severe

Total muscle **rupture**. There may be complete loss of muscle function. The injury needs at least a 6 week recovery and may require surgery.

Correct treatment during the first three days after the injury is critical for a quick recovery:

- **compression** – bandage the injury to reduce swelling
- cold – apply ice wrapped in a towel every eight hours for 15–20 minutes or until the area feels numb
- rest – any movement that causes pain means the injury is getting worse.

compression bandage

njuries from these activities cause
ne most hospital visits for
hildren.

	Per centage of visits
ycling	26.2
ootball	11.3
ollerskating and rollerblading	6.5
asketball	6.3
occer	6.0
rampolining	6.0
kateboarding	5.1
Cricket	3.7
Netball	3.7
Rugby	3.6

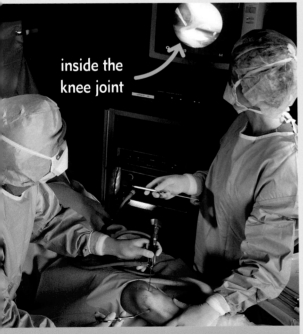

inside the
knee joint

Some torn ligaments are repaired
by surgery. Ligament injuries can
make joints unstable.

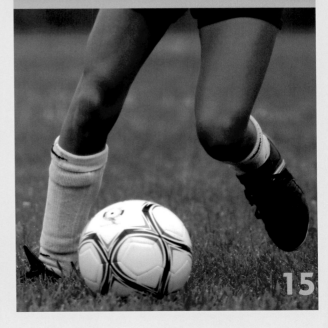

Knee injuries are common when
there are sudden sideways
movements, or hits to the side of
the legs.

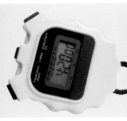

Measuring Fitness

Measure how your body responds to exercise, and test how fit you are.

Note: Ask an adult to help with this procedure.

You will need:

- stopwatch, or watch with a second hand
- pen and paper
- chair.

What to do:

1 Measure and record your pulse (heart rate). Place two fingers on the side of your neck, just under your jaw. Count the number of beats you feel in 10 seconds, and then multiply that number by six to calculate beats per minute.

2 Measure and record your breathing rate. Count the number of breaths in 10 seconds, and then multiply that number by six to calculate breaths per minute.

3 Step onto and off the chair at a steady pace for three minutes. Ask someone to hold the chair still.

4 Immediately repeat steps 1 and 2.

5 Repeat step 3, rest for three minutes, and then repeat steps 1 and 2 again.

The lower your pulse and breathing rates are after exercise, the fitter you are. How long did it take for your breathing and pulse rates to return to resting levels?

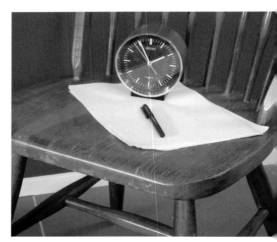

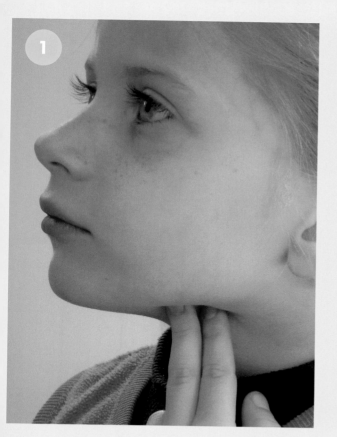

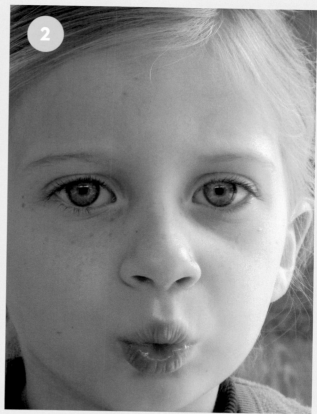

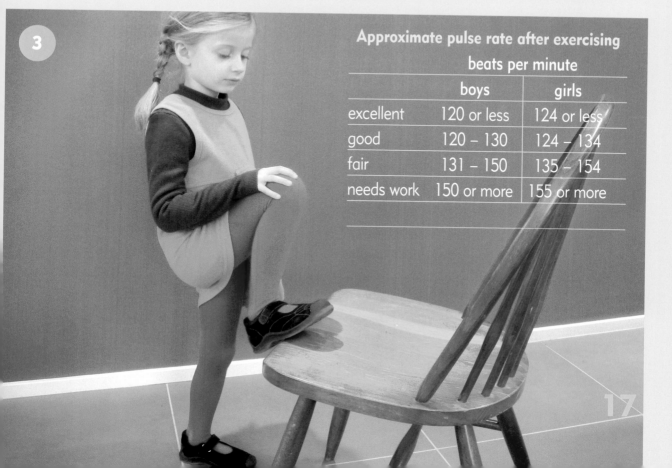

Approximate pulse rate after exercising beats per minute		
	boys	girls
excellent	120 or less	124 or less
good	120 – 130	124 – 134
fair	131 – 150	135 – 154
needs work	150 or more	155 or more

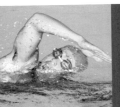

Swim Training

Training gives swimmers the speed, endurance, skill and focus they need to compete.

Typical training

For **elite** swimmers, a training session lasts about two hours. There may be 6–12 sessions each week.

A session begins with a warm-up of stretching and slow swimming. This is followed by laps – sometimes fast, sometimes slow. A swimmer training for a 1 500 metre race may swim more than 30 miles each week.

Coaches correct stroke **technique** and oversee start and turn **drills**. The session ends with a cool-down swim. Swimmers also do weight training to build strength.

Equipment

Swimmers use equipment while they are training in the pool. Kickboards help them focus on leg movements. Pull buoys held between the legs stop their feet from kicking, so swimmers can concentrate on arm movements. Paddles are used to strengthen arms and shoulders by providing resistance against the water.

Ready to compete

Swimmers change their training routines as a competition approaches. The **tapering** period rests the body and conserves energy for racing. Swimmers focus on skills and race **tactics**, and build confidence for the race.

GO FACT!

FIRST AND ONLY

Swimmer Shane Gould was 15 years old when she became the only person – male or female – to hold every world freestyle record from 100 m to 1 500 m simultaneously.

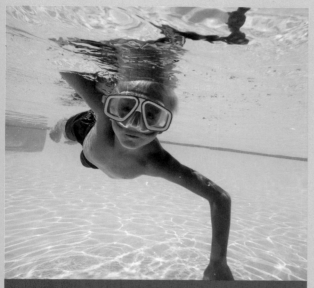

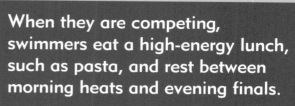

When they are competing, swimmers eat a high-energy lunch, such as pasta, and rest between morning heats and evening finals.

Underwater swimming was once an Olympic sport. Frenchman Charles de Vendeville swam 60 metres in one breath to win at the 1900 Olympic Games.

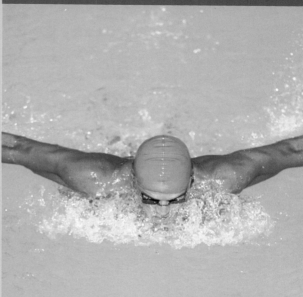

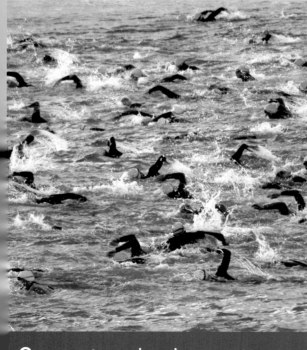

Swimmers wear goggles to protect their eyes from chlorine in the water.

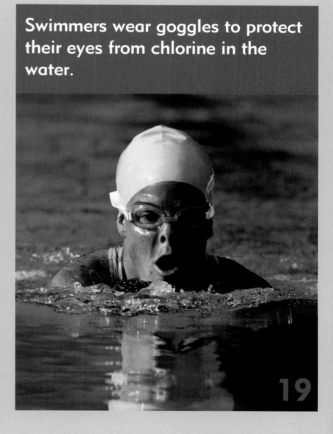

Open-water swimming events are held in rivers, lakes and oceans.

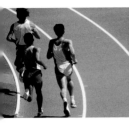

Running

Running seems like a simple activity, but it is actually a complex cycle of movements. The running cycle is divided into two phases.

Stance phase

The stance phase begins as the heel strikes the ground. In the midstance position, the foot bears all the body's weight. The toes push away from the ground at take-off, driving the runner up and forward.

Swing phase

The swing phase describes the leg's movement off the ground. After take-off, the foot swings forward as the thigh moves forward and the knee extends. The leg straightens before the foot hits the ground to begin the stance phase again.

The running cycle

As one leg moves through the stance phase, the other leg moves through the swing phase. Arm movements balance and lift the runner. The arms are bent at right angles, matching the forward movement of the opposite leg.

Most elite runners breathe in time with their running cycle – they breathe in for two steps and out for two steps.

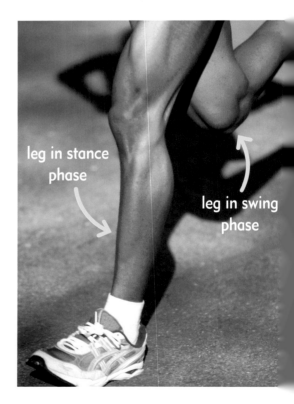

leg in stance phase

leg in swing phase

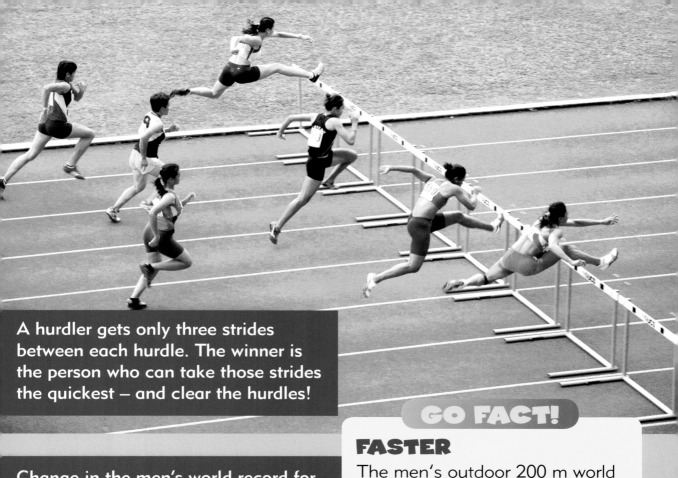

A hurdler gets only three strides between each hurdle. The winner is the person who can take those strides the quickest — and clear the hurdles!

Change in the men's world record for running one mile (1·6 kilometres).

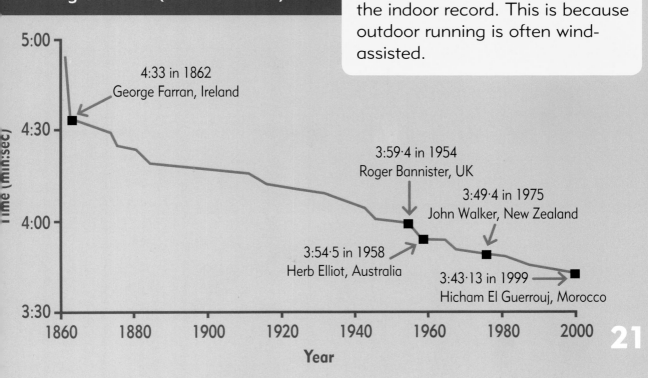

4:33 in 1862
George Farran, Ireland

3:59·4 in 1954
Roger Bannister, UK

3:49·4 in 1975
John Walker, New Zealand

3:54·5 in 1958
Herb Elliot, Australia

3:43·13 in 1999
Hicham El Guerrouj, Morocco

Time (min:sec)

Year

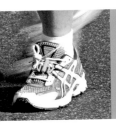

The Marathon

The marathon is the longest running race in athletics.

The first Olympic marathon was held in Athens in 1896. It was based on the **legend** of Pheidippides, a Greek soldier who ran approximately 25 miles carrying a message from the town of Marathon to Athens in 490 BC.

At the 1908 Olympic Games, the distance was set at 26 miles, which was the distance from Windsor Castle to the stadium in London.

In the race

Marathon runners usually run the first 18 miles at a steady pace. They then increase speed towards the finish line. Whoever leads the race must push into the wind, so the runner in first place often tries to convince other runners to lead.

Runners **dehydrate** due to sweating and breathing. During a race, marathon runners consume sports drinks, which contain **carbohydrate** for energy and salts to help the body absorb fluids.

Recovery

After the race, runners drink and eat to replace fluids and energy. Muscle soreness is normal after a marathon, but stretching within 20 minutes of finishing helps to reduce pain.

Most runners only compete in two or three marathons each year, to give themselves time for training and recovery.

GO FACT!
DID YOU KNOW?

At the 1904 Olympic Games, American Fred Lorz took a lift in a car before finishing the marathon on foot as the winner. He was disqualified.

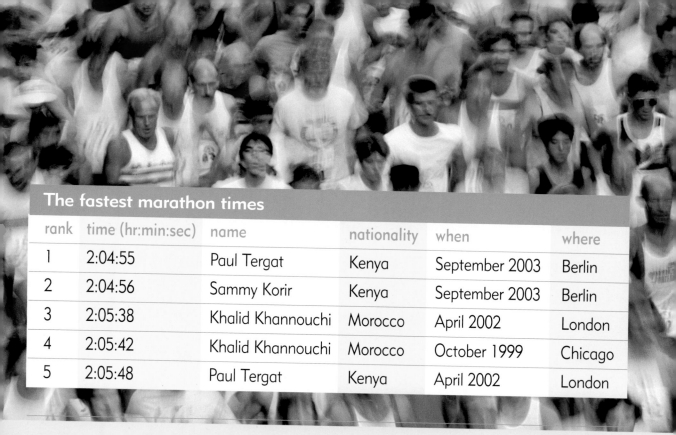

The fastest marathon times

rank	time (hr:min:sec)	name	nationality	when	where
1	2:04:55	Paul Tergat	Kenya	September 2003	Berlin
2	2:04:56	Sammy Korir	Kenya	September 2003	Berlin
3	2:05:38	Khalid Khannouchi	Morocco	April 2002	London
4	2:05:42	Khalid Khannouchi	Morocco	October 1999	Chicago
5	2:05:48	Paul Tergat	Kenya	April 2002	London

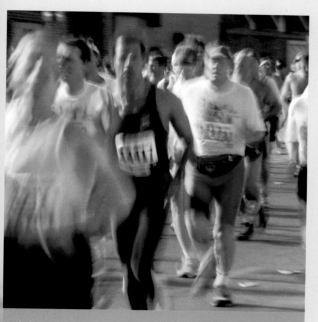

More than 35 000 runners compete in the New York City Marathon, the world's largest annual marathon.

At the annual Man versus Horse Marathon in Wales, runners compete against riders on horseback. In 27 years, a runner has only won once.

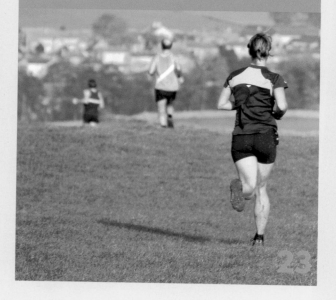

23

An Athlete's Diet

Athletes eat healthy foods that their bodies quickly store as energy.

Eating to win

Carbohydrates, such as bread, pasta, cereal, fruit and vegetables, are the best sources of energy. The human body can only store limited carbohydrates, so most athletes eat five to six meals each day. A top-level football player needs about 5–8 grams of carbohydrate per kilogram of body weight each day.

To get energy when they need it, athletes eat a lot of **portable** foods, such as cereal bars, fruit, dried fruit, juice and milk.

Athletes also need protein, fats, vitamins and minerals. Iron is important for rowers, so their diet includes sources of iron, such as lean red meat, chicken and green vegetables.

On your mark!

On competition days, athletes eat low-fat, high-carbohydrate meals. They eat 2–4 hours before an event.

Athletes who play a seasonal sport, such as hockey or baseball, eat less during the off-season to match the decrease in training.

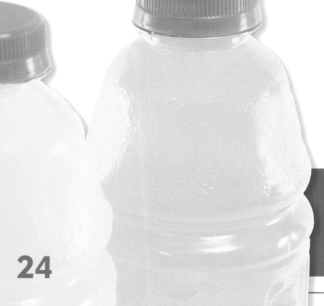

Sports drinks contain about half the sugar that soft drinks contain.

Triathletes fit their meals and snacks around 2–3 daily training sessions.

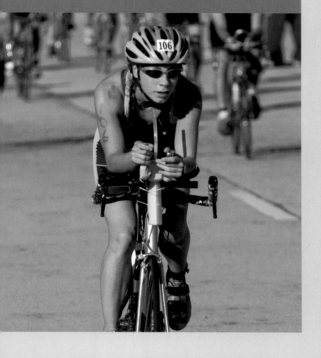

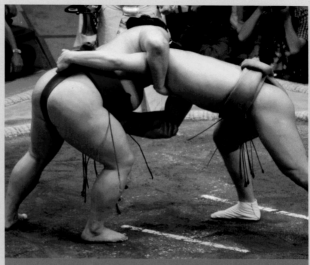

Sumo wrestlers eat healthy food — a lot of it! To reach a weight of more than 200 kilograms, they eat huge meals and then sleep, so that most of the energy from the food is stored as fat.

Each of these snacks gives 50 grams of carbohydrate

- 800 – 1 000 mL sports drink
- 3 medium-sized pieces of fruit
- salad roll
- 2 cereal bars
- 2 x 200 g cartons of yoghurt
- bowl of cereal with low-fat milk
- bowl of fruit salad with 100 g yoghurt
- 250 – 350 mL smoothie
- 3 slices toast.

People who play snow sports need plenty of liquids. They lose fluids via sweating and from breathing cold, dry air.

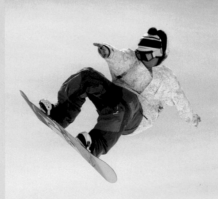

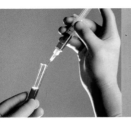

Drugs in Sport

Some athletes take performance-enhancing drugs to gain an advantage over their competitors. This is illegal.

Some drugs are legal for athletes, such as those for treating injuries. Others are banned because they improve performance and are dangerous to an athlete's health. Taking these drugs is called doping – it is a way of cheating.

The World Anti-Doping Agency promotes the fight against doping in sport. National anti-doping agencies regularly test athletes to find out if they are taking banned drugs. Testing **deters** athletes from cheating and detects athletes who are doping.

Banned for life?

An athlete who fails a doping test may be banned from their sport for life. For example, former world champion Australian weightlifter Sergo Chakhoyan received a two-year ban for failing a doping test in 2001. When he failed a second test in 2005, he was banned for life.

A life ban is a very harsh penalty. It ends a sporting career, which is often an athlete's source of income. Some people claim the doping tests are not reliable.

On the other hand, athletes know the penalties for doping, and most sports give athletes a second chance if they fail one test. Some athletes continue to take drugs even after they are caught. This is why the penalty is so harsh.

A sports performance should only depend on an athlete's talent, determination, courage and honesty – not on drugs.

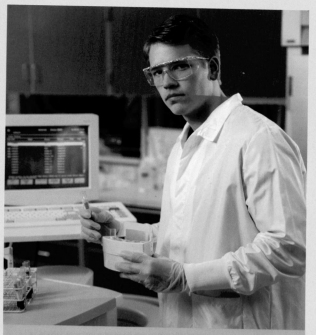

There is no limit to the number of times an athlete can be tested each year.

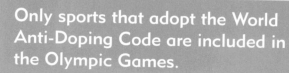

Only sports that adopt the World Anti-Doping Code are included in the Olympic Games.

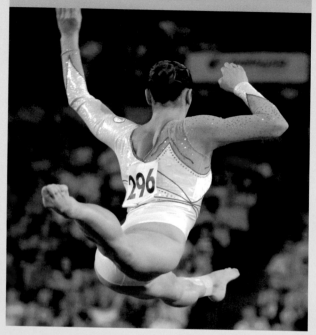

Cyclists used caffeine, cocaine and alcohol in the nineteenth century.

Between 1983 and 2005, athletes failed only 32 of the 3 475 doping tests conducted at the World Athletics Championships.

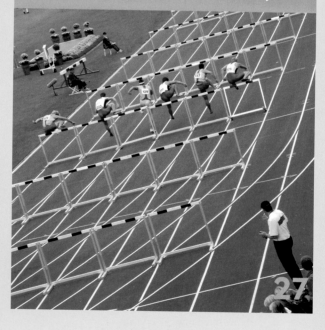

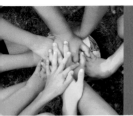

Be Fit!

Fitness increases physical strength, improves mental health and builds friendships.

For the body

Moderate exercise for 30 minutes each day, five days a week, benefits your health.

Being fit reduces the risk of heart disease, high blood pressure and diabetes. It increases the body's energy levels and helps maintain a healthy weight.

Exercise creates strong bones and strengthens the **immune system**, so the body is more able to stay healthy.

For the mind

Regular exercise helps to improve mental **wellbeing**.

When people become depressed, they often have no energy or motivation. They become less active. People who isolate themselves from other people are at greater risk of developing depression and take longer to recover.

For friends

Exercising is a great way to meet people and make new friends.

Joining a team or club gives people a sense of belonging, and may bring lifelong friendships.

Some people try many sports before they find the one that is right for them.

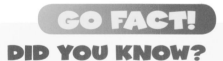

GO FACT!

DID YOU KNOW?

People who exercise intensely and regularly may add more than three years to their lives.

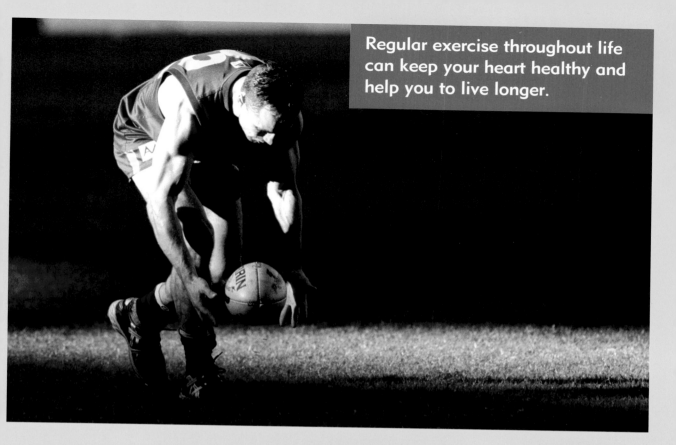

Regular exercise throughout life can keep your heart healthy and help you to live longer.

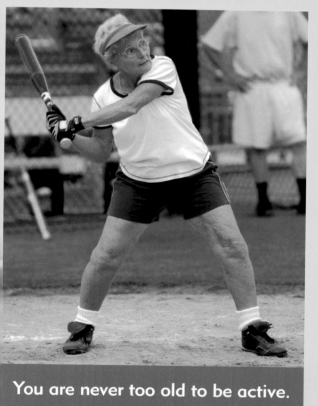

You are never too old to be active.

In the UK, the most popular physical activities for males are walking, golf and swimming. The most popular activities for females are walking, aerobics and swimming.

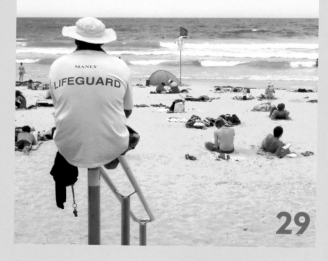

 # Oldest World Records

event	name, country	record set	
1 men's 50 m pistol shooting	Aleksandr Melentiev, USSR	20 July 1980	
2 women's 800 m athletics	Jarmila Kratochvílová, Czechoslovakia	26 July 1983	
3 women's 400 m athletics	Marita Koch, East Germany	6 October 1985	
4 women's 4 x 100 m relay athletics	East German team	6 October 1985	
5 men's discus throw	Jürgen Schult, East Germany	6 June 1986	
6 men's hammer throw	Yuriy Sedykh, USSR	30 August 1986	

Glossary

aerobic (adjective) (means 'with oxygen') relating to exercise which improves the use of oxygen by the body

anaerobic (adjective) (means 'without oxygen') relating to exercise in which the body's muscles produce energy without oxygen

carbohydrate (noun) any of a large group of substances, including sugars, which are a source of energy for animals and plants

compression (noun) the action of compressing; pressing or squeezing together

dehydrate (verb) to lose water from the body

deter (verb) to discourage someone from doing something, often through fear of the results

drill (noun) an activity which practises a skill, often by repeating the same thing several times

elastic (adjective) able to stretch and be returned to its original shape or size

elite (adjective) belonging to an elite, which is a group of people regarded as the best

immune system (noun) the body's organs and glands that allow it to protect itself against disease

inflamed (adjective) red, painful and swollen

legend (noun) a very old story, which may not be true

ligament (noun) a strong, flexible strip of tissue that connects bones

nutrient (noun) any substance which plants or animals need to live and grow

perspiration (noun) sweat; the process of perspiring

portable (adjective) able to be easily carried

rupture (verb) to burst, break or tear

skeletal muscle (noun) a muscle attached to a bone

tactic (noun) a planned way of doing something

tapering (adjective) becoming smaller or less frequent

technique (noun) a way of doing an activity which needs skill

tissue (noun) a group or layer of cells that have a similar function

wellbeing (noun) the state of feeling healthy and happy

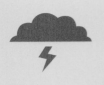

Index

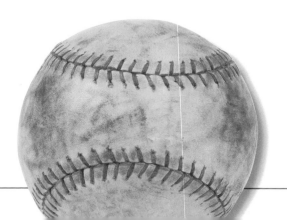